Synesthesia.

The Fascinating World
of Blended Senses.

Synesthesia and
Types of Synesthesia Explained.

by

Lyndsay Leatherdale

Published by IMB Publishing 2013

Acknowledgements

Thank you to my interviewees, who generously shared their experiences with me for this book: Joanne, Chris, Melissa, Sheila and Nicole, and to the many other people who got in touch on Twitter to share their own synesthesia stories.

For a list of the books and websites I consulted during the course of my research, please go to the Resources chapter at the end of this book.

Table of Contents

Table Of Contents

Foreword

Synesthesia is a fascinating condition. We often talk about synesthetes (the name given to people with synesthesia) 'tasting colours' and 'seeing music', but as you'll see in this book, it's a lot more complicated than that.

Synesthesia has long been associated with creativity and the arts. It's been a huge gift to musicians such as Stevie Wonder (who, despite his blindness, is able to 'see' music as colour), and it is thought that Beethoven and Schubert may also have been synesthetes.

Many famous painters across history have had synaesthesia. Probably the most famous is Wassily Kandinsky, whose bold and colourful abstract paintings were inspired by music. As a child, he heard a hissing sound coming from his paint-box, and later learned that this was because looking at colours made him hear sound.

This also worked in reverse, meaning that listening to music inspired his paintings. After attending a Wagner concert in Moscow in 1910, he said:

"I saw all my colours in spirit, before my eyes. Wild, almost crazy lines were sketched in front of me. " Wassily Kandinsky

Other famous synesthetes include actor Geoffrey Rush (who sees the days of the week as colours), musician Billy Joel (who sees vowels and consonants as different colours) and author of Chocolat, Joanne Harris (who senses colours as scents).

I asked Joanne whether synesthesia had affected her writing. 'Until very recently, I thought it was normal,' she said. This sums up the experiences of many people with synesthesia: it's a part of their everyday life, and they may not even realise that they're seeing the world differently to everyone else.

In fact, for most people, synesthesia enhances their abilities and helps them to become successful in their chosen field. However, for a minority of people, synesthesia can have negative side effects. We will look at those, and what can be done to help, later in this book.

Whether you have synesthesia yourself, or are just curious about this extraordinary condition, this book is for you.

Chapter 1) About Synesthesia

We take a look at how synesthesia is defined by neuroscientists and how common it is. We also examine the history of how we've come to understand synesthesia.

1) What is Synesthesia?

The Definition of Synesthesia

Synesthesia is a neurological condition- meaning that it exists in the brain and nervous system. People with synesthesia experience their senses in an unusual way; input to one sense will lead to a response from a different sense.

For example, it might mean that hearing a sound will make you see a colour; or tasting something could make you hear music. This is sometimes described as a 'blending' of the senses.

The Definition of Synesthete

A synesthete is the word used to describe someone with synesthesia. This is a useful term, because synesthetes often feel that they have special skills and ways of seeing the world, and so do not want to be called 'sufferers' or 'patients', which are terms we would perhaps use for other neurological conditions.

The Features of Synesthesia

The neurologist Richard Cytowic is perhaps the best-known expert on synesthesia. In his book, 'Synesthesia: A Union of the Senses' (1989), he identified five key features of the condition.

8

1. **It is involuntary and automatic** – this means that it is not something that you can choose to have. Your brain does the work without you even noticing.

2. **Synesthetic experiences are consistent and generic** - they are the same every time you experience them.

3. **It is highly memorable** – people tend to remember their synesthetic experiences, rather than forget them or not really notice them.

4. **It has affect** – this means that it creates an emotional response. Synesthetes don't feel neutrally about their synesthesia; it matters to them. Synesthesia triggers the emotions.

In his original book, Cytowic added a fifth feature of synesthesia, which was that it is 'spatially extended', meaning that synesthetes experience their senses as though they're in a specific place, rather than in their brains. So they may hear a synesthetic sound coming from a certain direction, or look at a synesthetic colour as if it's appearing outside their body.

However, as he researched further, Cytowic realised that this only described some synesthetes. Writing with David Eagleman, Cytowic later said that there were two types of synesthetes:

1. **Localizers** – people whose synesthesia is 'spatially extended', as in the examples above.

2. **Non-Localizers**, who don't experience synesthesia in this way.

Non-localizers are in fact more common.

2) The History of Synesthesia

Synesthesia has always existed. There is evidence of people writing about seeing music as colour in ancient Greece. However, we only began to understand it as a condition about 200 years ago.

Doctors and scientists began to take an interest in synesthesia in the early 1800s, and the first study into synesthesia, which looked at the experiences of 73 synesthetes, took place in 1871.

However, it was not until around 1980 that scientists really began to understand synesthesia. As interest grew in cognitive science (the study of processes in the brain and how we experience them), synesthesia became an important clue to how the brain works. So, synesthetes have probably only been able to put a name to their condition for 100 years; and even then, few people would have known about synesthesia.

Much of the research contained in this book was only done in the last thirty years. There are many aspects of the condition that remain mysterious, but as you will see, we now understand more about the causes of synesthesia, and the forms that it takes.

Neuroscientists are now so interested in synesthesia that synesthetes can take part in any number of research projects on the subject. Most famously, the Synesthesia Battery, run by David Eagleman, is a website containing a range of tests that synesthetes (or people who suspect they have synesthesia) can take. The data is then made available to researchers studying the condition.

You can find this at http://synesthete.org.

3) How Common is Synesthesia?

One of the reasons that people find synesthesia fascinating is because it's so hard to understand and study. The problem is, we're not entirely sure how common it is: few people with the condition tell their doctor. Some don't even realise that they have synesthesia in the first place, and others diagnose themselves with the condition, and don't feel the need to visit any medical professionals because they have nothing that they want to have 'cured' or 'treated.'

This means that different neuroscientists estimate that synesthesia affects between one in 2,000 and one in 20 people. That's a huge range. What these figures show is that it's common to have some kind of synesthetic experience in your life, perhaps only one thing, such as associating a day of the week with a colour. But it's far more rare to have the more complex forms of synesthesia, which have a strong effect on how you feel on a day-to-day basis.

The numbers appear to be growing, but we are not sure if that's because more people are actually getting synesthesia, or just because more people are being diagnosed with the condition.

What we do understand is that some forms of synesthesia are more common than others. Research by Sean Day, a linguist and synesthete, shows that the most common forms of synesthesia are as follows:

Type of Synesthesia	% Frequency
Graphemes (letters) to Colour	62.51
Ticker-Tape (Sound to vision)	21.91
Musical notes to Flavours	19.23
Sounds to Colour	14.72
Personalities to Touch	8.92
Mirror Touch (Other people's sensations)	8.7
Phonemes (speech) to Colour	6.66
Flavours to Colour	6.23
Smells to Touch	5.91
Pain to Colour	5.26

Data from http://daysyn.com/types-of-syn © Sean Day 2013-08-20

It's worth pointing out that the percentages here are not of the general population, but of all synesthetes. So for example, Graphemes to Colour synesthesia is by far the most common form of the disease, affecting 62.5 per cent of all synesthetes.
In the next chapter, we will take a closer look at the different types of synesthesia, both common and rare.

Chapter 1 Summary
- Synesthesia affects between one in twenty and one in two thousand people.
- You can't choose or learn to have synesthesia: it's involuntary.

- It creates memorable experiences with emotional impact.
- Synesthetic experiences remain the same over time.
- You may feel that your synesthesia happens outside your body, but you may also feel that it happens inside your head.
- We have only really begun to understand synesthesia in the last 30 years.

Chapter 2) Forms of Synesthesia

Synesthesia isn't just one condition:
it's actually a cluster of experiences that are
linked by sensory cross-over.
In this chapter, we take a look at the
most common forms of synesthesia.

1) How the Forms are Sorted

There are many different forms of synesthesia (probably more than 60 in total), some of which are extremely rare.

As you already know, synesthesia is when input to one sense leads to a response from a different sense. Therefore, for the purposes of this chapter, we will group the different forms of synesthesia by the input sense - for example, if hearing a sound makes you see colour, your form of synesthesia would be in the section on hearing.

After each definition, we have also provided the frequency percentage from Sean Day's research; as with the previous chapter, this is the percentage of all synesthetes that have this form of synesthesia, rather than the percentage of all the people in the world.

It's worth noting that around half of all synesthetes will have more than one form of synesthesia, and so may not experience their synesthesia as a distinct form, but will rather feel that they have a cluster of synesthetic reactions.

Finally, there are forms of synesthesia that aren't listed here, because they are so rare and so don't show up in the frequency tables. If you have blended senses but don't see your particular mix here, it doesn't mean that it's not synesthesia; it's just that it's a rare form and hasn't yet been documented.

2) Language

Grapheme to Colour Synesthesia

Associating letters or numbers with different colours as you read them. This is by far the most common form of synesthesia, and may affect up to one per cent of the world's population.
Frequency: 62.5%

Phoneme to Colours Synesthesia

Phonemes are the individual sounds that make up words (such as 'll' or 's' or 'ck'). Parents may be familiar with these sounds from teaching phonics to their children when they're learning to read. In this form of synesthesia, the individual sounds that make up a word are associated with different colours, so a whole word may be multi-coloured.
Frequency: 6.7%

Grapheme Personification Synesthesia

Numbers, letters, days of the month and other common elements of life are associated with personalities, especially when reading.
Frequency: 2.69%

Lexeme to Flavour (Lexical-Gustatory) Synesthesia

Certain words are experienced as flavours.
Frequency: 0.2%

Lexeme to Odour Synesthesia

Words are experienced as smells.
Frequency: 0.4%

Ordinal-Linguistic Personification

In this form of synesthesia, well-known sequences, such as days of the week, months or numbers are experienced as personalities.
In one of the earliest studies of synesthesia, Théodore Flournoy quoted a woman he called Madame L., who experienced numbers as distinct personalities:

"1, 2, 3 are children without fixed personalities; they play together. 4 is a good peaceful woman, absorbed by down-to-earth occupations and who takes pleasure in them. 5 is a young man, ordinary and common in his tastes and appearance, but extravagant and self-centred. 6 is a young man of 16 or 17, very well brought-up, polite, gentle, agreeable in appearance, and with upstanding tastes; average intelligence; orphan..." Madame L.

After number 10, the numbers had no personalities for her.
Frequency: 0.1%

3) Vision

Mirror Touch Synesthesia

Mirror Touch is a little different to other forms of synesthesia, in that synesthetes seem to be reproducing the same feeling, rather than having an entirely different one.

Sufferers (this is one of the rare types of synesthesia that tend to be seen as negative) can feel sensations that they see other people experiencing. So, for example, they may watch a violent act in a film, and feel the pain themselves.

"If I see someone else get hurt, I feel a sensation in my own body. It even works if someone's describing an injury: my mind replays it as if I'm the one getting hurt, and I can feel every part of it."
Chris

15

Frequency: 8.7%

Vision to Sound Synesthesia

These synesthetes hear sounds when they see certain things, often colours.

"Colours have sounds and styles to them, if I'm bombarded by a lot of really bright colours, it's bit of a cacophony and can get quite loud. I tend, in my décor preferences, to like neural colours, as they are quieter." Nicole.
Frequency: 0.32%

Vision to Smells Synesthesia or Vision to Flavours Synesthesia

These synesthetes find that certain things they see trigger smells or flavours.
Frequency: 0.1 - 0.3%

Vision to Kinetics Synesthesia or Vision to Touch Synesthesia

In this form of synesthesia, certain sights trigger a feeling of movement or being touched by an object. These synesthetes sometimes describe sensations such as being struck by a wave or being punched. Other feelings are more pleasant, such as a light breeze or a vibration.
Frequency: 0.97% (Vision to Touch unknown)

Vision to Temperature Synesthesia

Certain sights make the synesthete feel sensations of warmth or cold. This is most commonly triggered by colour.

Frequency: 1.93%

4) Touch

Touch to Temperature Synesthesia

Touch is perceived as a certain temperature on the skin. Frequency: 3.1%

Pain to Colour Synesthesia

For some, physical sensation is associated with colour. Most commonly, this happens when the person is in pain, but it can also occur with any touch.

In a 1913 study in the Journal of Abnormal Psychology, Isador Coriat described a patient who recognised different types of pain, and associated a colour with each:

*"Each type of pain produced its individual and invariable colour, for instance: Hollow pain, blue colour; sore pain, red colour; deep headache, vivid scarlet; superficial headache, white colour; shooting neuralgic pain, white color."*Marianne
Frequency: 5.26% (1.1% for Touch to Colour Synesthesia).

Touch to Flavour Synesthesia or Touch to Smell Synesthesia

These synesthetes experience different tastes and odours when they touch different surfaces. For example, a person may have different associations from touching skin, silk, sandpaper or wood. Frequency: 0.3 – 0.4%

17

Touch to Emotion Synesthesia

In this very rare form of synesthesia, people experience strong emotions from touching different surfaces.

In an article in the Daily Mail in August 2013, one 27-year old woman reported to feeling very strong emotions from these encounters:

"Touching corduroy left her confused, leather aroused feelings of receiving criticism, multi-coloured toothpaste made her feel anxious, wax made her feel embarrassed, paracetamol tablets left her feeling jealous and different grades of sandpaper made her feel either guilt, relief, or as if she was telling a white lie." Peter
Frequency: Unknown.

5) Taste

Flavour to Colour Synesthesia

Tastes are experienced as different colours.
Frequency: 6.2%

Flavour to Touch Synesthesia or Flavour to Temperature Synesthesia

Tastes are experienced as physical sensations (such as tickling) or textures (such as prickly). More rarely (0.1% of cases), synesthetes can experience flavours as different temperatures.
Frequency: 0.5%

Flavour to Sound Synesthesia

Tastes are experienced as different sounds – for example, you might think that fish tastes like a clarinet.
Frequency: 0.3%

6) Sound

Sound to Colour (Chromesthesia)

This is one of the most common forms of synesthesia, in which different qualities of sound are experienced as distinct colours. According to Richard Cytowic, this is a bit like watching a firework display, with explosions of colour being triggered by various sounds, and then gradually fading away.

Many famous musicians and composers have this form of synesthesia, such as country musician John Mayer and composer Franz Liszt.

More rarely, synesthetes can perceive specific musical notes as colour. For these people, chords or scales may also have a colour, or may be a blend of the colours that come from each of their notes.

*"I hear colour, and musical keys produce an overall hue that I can see, which washes over and slightly tints any visuals, i.e. the key of C major is a bright blue, E flat minor is a sort of jaguar green."*Nicole
Frequency: 14.72% (Musical Sounds to Colours: 0.1%)

Sound to Vision (Ticker Tape) Synesthesia

This is distinct from sound to colour synesthesia, as it means that the synesthete receives visions of objects, patterns, textures or shapes. For many, it seems to flash before their eyes; many people

with this form of synesthesia report seeing subtitles of the words they're hearing.
Frequency: 21.9%

Sound to Temperature Synesthesia or Sound to Touch Synesthesia

It's relatively common for synesthetes to experience sounds as different temperatures. Some people also experience sounds as textures or sensations, but this is so rare that we can't provide a percentage frequency.
Frequency: 3.9%

Sound to Flavours Synesthesia and Sound to Smell Synesthesia

Similar to Lexical-Gustatory Synesthesia, this form of the condition makes people perceive sounds as tastes or odours. This, of course, can mean that certain sounds are extremely unpleasant because they're associated with nasty odours or tastes; but also that some are wonderful.

Synesthete James Wannerton, interviewed for the Wellcome Trust, says that because of his sound to flavour synesthesia, he doesn't seem to get as hungry as other people, because the sounds themselves satisfy him!
Frequency: 0.5 – 0.9%

Musical Notes to Flavours Synesthesia

Perhaps surprisingly, it is more common for musicians to link specific notes to certain flavours, rather than general sounds.
Frequency: 19.2%

Sound to Kinetics Synesthesia

Here, sounds are associated with the sensation of moving, even if the synesthete is standing still. Some synesthetes describe this as being hit by a wave or an earthquake.
Frequency: 1.5%

7) Smell

Smell to Touch Synesthesia and Smell to Temperature Synesthesia

In smell to touch synesthesia, people associate certain odours with physical sensations, such as texture or pressure.
Less commonly, some people experience smells as different temperatures.
Frequency: 5.9% (0.5% for smell to temperature)

Smell to Flavour Synesthesia

The sense of smell is linked to how we taste foods in most people, but for certain synesthetes, an odour can trigger a flavour that's completely separate from the substance that they can smell. For example, it's perfectly normal to smell fish and to get an impression of how it will taste, but a synesthete may perhaps smell fish and taste strawberries.
Frequency: 0.5%

Smell to Sound Synesthesia and Smell to Vision Synesthesia

These are both rare forms of synesthesia, in which an odour can trigger the synesthete to experience sounds or colours respectively.

"I have always been aware of 'seeing' smells. It's not a physical sight of them, more the shape they take in my brain as I perceive them.

*For example, if I think of my favourite perfume - Cashmere Mist by Donna Karen -it is a soft, powdery, clean fragrance that spirals continually, getting wider as it does so. The smell of freshly made Morning Glory tea is flat, regular lines, gently floating on top of each other. Lemon is different sizes of spheres bobbing about, and the smell of my kitten's head is fine tendrils reaching out around me. "*Melissa

Frequency: 0.1%

8) Emotion

Emotion to Colour Synesthesia

For some synesthetes, emotions make them see colours. This way of seeing the world is quite commonly found in popular culture, such as experiencing 'blue' moods or seeing 'red' when we're angry. However, for genuine synesthetes, this experience will be much more vivid and consistent across time.

Frequency: 1.93%

Emotion to Odour Synesthesia and Emotion to Flavour Synesthesia

For these synesthetes, emotions will often be experienced as odours or tastes.

Some people with the condition report smelling an emotion before they feel it consciously.

Frequency: 0.1 – 0.2%

Emotion to Sound Synesthesia

22

In this rare form of the condition, emotions are experienced as sounds or music. For some people, this can be extremely overwhelming, especially when emotions are strongly negative. Frequency: 0.1%

9) Other Synesthetic Inputs

Kinetics

Kinetics are the sense of movement.
When the synesthete moves, they can experience sound or see colours, or can feel that certain movements have a personality; for example, a brisk walk might be bossy.

Alternatively, the same effects may arise from watching movement from the outside, whether that is a person or an object, such as a car or a swing.
Frequency: 0.1 – 1.0%

Personality

Some synesthetes can associate different colours, sounds, smells or sensations with the personalities of people they meet.

When this involves colour, it can take the form of an 'aura' floating around the person in question.
Frequency: 0.1 – 8.9%

Object Personification

For a synesthete, a completely inanimate object (such as a chair, glass or rug) can have a personality, and this can be as complex and detailed as a well-known friend.

This can lead to very negative associations with certain objects, causing the synesthete a great deal of distress. Or, in rare cases, it can take the form of objectum sexuality, which means that the synesthete develops a sometimes intense sexual attraction to an object.
Frequency: 2.2% (Objectum Sexuality: unknown)

23

Orgasm

While we're on the subject of sex, it's fairly common for synesthetes to experience a blending of the senses during orgasm. The most common synesthetic experience here is encountering tastes during orgasm (5.9% frequency), but some synesthetes also see colour (0.1%).

Number

We have already looked at the ways in which synesthetes can have an altered visual sense of how numbers look. However, there are other synesthetic experiences around numbers, which involve the concept of the quantity, rather than the written number.

For example, certain synesthetes have spatial sequence synesthesia around numbers, which means that they see numbers as existing in certain physical locations, or at certain distances away from the synesthete. This can also work for other sequences too, such as the alphabet or days of the week.

Time, too, can be perceived synesthetically, sometimes as colours or sounds.
Frequency: 2.2 – 4.0%

Chapter 2 Summary
- There are many different types of synesthesia, each with a different input and output sense, including taste, vision, language, smell and movement.
- Over 50 per cent of synesthetes have more than one type of synesthesia.
- By far the most common form of synesthesia is grapheme to colour synesthesia, meaning that 62.5 per cent of all synesthetes associate letters with colours.

Chapter 3) Who Gets Synesthesia?

Synesthesia tends to stay with you
for your whole life. We look at the factors that
make it more likely to appear, and the
ways in which synesthesia can be 'acquired'
later in life.

1) Genetics

Synesthesia is mostly genetically inherited – in other words, passed
from parent to child. Research shows that around 40 per cent of
people with synesthesia have a parent who also has the condition.

Even if a parent doesn't have synesthesia but a child does, it could
still have been genetically inherited, because people can carry
synesthesia genes without experiencing any symptoms.

Julian Asher of the Welcome Trust Centre for Genetics and Simon
Baron-Cohen of the University of Cambridge have conducted a
study of 43 families that have members who have synesthesia. They
identified three particular chromosomes that carry synesthesia.

These chromosomes carried genes that governed the development
of the cerebral cortex, the correct development of neurons and
electrical signalling in the brain (see Chapter 4 for more information
on how the brain works).

The location of the genes for synesthesia suggested a strong link to
autism, and it is common for people with autism to experience some
of the symptoms of synesthesia. However, this does not mean that
all synesthetes are autistic, but that the two conditions have some
common traits.

The more genetic research that is conducted into synesthesia, the
more scientists understand that it is a very complex condition that

can be inherited through a wide variety of routes. This perhaps accounts for the many different ways in which people experience synesthesia.

2) Gender

More women than men tend to have synesthesia, but the bias towards women is not as strong as we once thought.

Researchers have often assumed that synesthesia is carried on the X chromosome. The X and Y chromosomes determine whether we are male or female; females have two 'X' chromosomes and men have an 'X' and a 'Y'.

This means that there are some conditions that women are more likely to get then men, because the genes for the disease are carried on the X chromosome and women get two of them.

Conversely, there are some conditions that only men get, such as certain forms of colour blindness, which are carried on the Y chromosome, and so are very rare in women.

However, the research by Simon Baron-Cohen, mentioned in the previous section, showed that synesthesia is not carried on the X chromosome, so it is now not clear why there are more female synesthetes than male ones. This could be connected to the very complex array of genes that govern synesthesia.

Women may also be more likely to report the condition, which would mean that synesthesia falsely appears to affect more women than men. This theory is supported by the fact that, as time goes on, we are noticing that a far greater proportion of men have synesthesia than we previously thought.

3) Age

Because synesthesia is genetically inherited, most synesthetes will have the condition all their lives. Many will report early memories that are connected to synesthetic experiences, even if they did not understand that they had the condition at that time.

The youngest reported case of synesthesia was a boy aged three, but it is likely that we only notice that children have synesthesia once their language skills become good enough to describe their experiences. They also need to begin to understand how others see the world, so that they can realise that their perceptions are different.

Some studies suggest that all infants under six months of age may see the world as a synesthete does. Research by Katie Wagner showed that babies of two and three months had the same strong associations between shape and colour that you would expect to see in a synesthetic adult. This disappears entirely by eight months of age.

This may point to synesthesia being a necessary phase in normal brain development.

4) Acquired Synesthesia

Some cases of synesthesia arise later in life, as the result of an illness or injury. This is called 'acquired' synesthesia, to distinguish it from the more common form of synesthesia, which is transmitted in our genes.

Brain Damage or Injury

In very rare conditions, people can develop synesthesia as a result of brain injury.

In 2013, doctors in Toronto documented only the second known case of a man who became a synesthete following a stroke. This patient found that many of his senses had become blended: colours evoked tastes and emotions, sounds became colours and tastes became colours too.

Dr Tom Schweitzer, a neuroscientist who studied the patient's responses using an MRI scanner, suggested that this case of synesthesia could have been caused by the brain trying to repair itself after damage done by the stroke, and making some unusual connections as it happened.

It also appeared that this synesthete's brain was responding to music and colour in unconventional areas of the brain. This could mean that the brain had found new ways of processing these inputs, after its more usual means had been damaged.

There have also been cases of synesthesia arising from damage done to the brain, brain tumours or spinal cord injury.

Blindness and Sensory Loss

Experiences similar to synesthesia are reported by people who became blind in later life.

Dr Jamie Ward of the University of Sussex has shown that newly blind people can start 'seeing' sound as colour very quickly. He suggests that losing one sense can activate pathways in the brain that have always existed (perhaps since infancy), but which aren't needed when all five senses are functioning.

His research shows that, if you artificially 'blind' someone by covering their eyes, they will start 'seeing' colour in this way after only a few days.

Narcotics

In some cases, taking hallucinogenic drugs such as LSD or mescalin can induce synesthesia-like symptoms. However, this is temporary and not common. More commonly, drug-users experience hallucinations that are not true synesthesia.

Epilepsy

A small number of epileptics experience synesthesia during seizures, when the electrical activity in the brain gives them sensory experiences, such as tastes or smells. This generally only lasts for the duration of the seizure.

Links to Other Conditions

The genetic study carried out by Julian Asher and Simon Baron-Cohen found that synesthesia was located on the same areas of the same chromosome as epilepsy, dyslexia and autism.

However, there is little evidence that synesthetes are more likely to also have these conditions; it's more likely that they all emerge at the same point in the brain's development, and share some common traits.

Some synesthetes feel that they are more likely to suffer from migraine, but once again, there is no strong link in the research. One of the issues here is that synesthesia covers such a wide variety of experiences and forms, to the extent that some people argue that it is actually a cluster of different but linked conditions.

Chapter 3 Summary
- Synesthesia is inherited through the genes of your parents.
- Neurological synesthesia is with you all your life.
- Women seem to be slightly more likely than men to get synesthesia, but it's not clear why or whether this is even the case.
- Synesthesia can be 'acquired' later in life through brain injury, drug use or epilepsy.
- It is linked to other conditions such as autism and epilepsy, but only in that it shares similar traits.

Chapter 4) The Neuroscience of Synesthesia

Neuroscience is the study of the brain and the nervous system. In this chapter, we will look at how the brain is constructed, and what differences we see in people with synesthesia.

1) The Brain

The human brain is divided into regions that are dedicated to a certain function. For example, the visual cortex governs seeing, the auditory cortex governs hearing and the motor cortex governs movement.

Therefore, when scientists study synesthesia, they are looking for ways in which these cortices can be connected to create a synesthetic experience. There is no one, clear theory of how synesthesia is created, and there are many different ways of experiencing synesthesia, but we will look at the main ideas in the field.

2) Cross-Activation

In some forms of synesthesia, such as grapheme to colour, the most common, the areas of the brain that interpret written text and colour are close together.

In normal brain development, a process called 'pruning' takes place, in which the regions of the brain become more separate over time (as we saw in Chapter 3, it's thought that babies' brains make connections in the same way as synesthetes, but that this is lost by eight months of age).

Cross-Activation theory suggests that this process fails to take place in synesthetes, and so they experience the characteristic 'blending' of different senses that continues from infancy.

This could also be true of lexical-gustatory synesthesia and taste to touch synesthesia. However, it would not explain all forms of synesthesia, because not all the cortices are next to each other.

3) Hyper-Excitable Brains

A 2011 study by researchers from Oxford University suggested that some brains are 'hyper-excitable'.

This study looked at the visual cortex of the brain, and found that, for synesthetes, it took much less stimulation to make the brains react than for people without synesthesia.

The researchers argue that this 'excitability' may lead to a blending of the senses. They tested their theory by applying weak magnetic currents to the brain from the outside of the head, and found that more stimulation can increase the intensity of synesthetic experiences.

However, once again, this research currently only covers visual synesthesia, and doesn't yet explain other forms.

4) Disinhibited Feedback

Some neuroscientists, such as Grossenbacher and Lovelace, argue that synesthesia may arise from a flaw in the way the brain talks to itself.

In normal circumstances, when your brain receives a piece of information (such as seeing a flower), a variety or areas of the brain 'light up' as they process it. A process called 'inhibition' ensures that the brain uses the correct balance of its areas to understand the information.

According to this theory, synesthetes lack this process of disinhibition, and so feel as though they are receiving feedback from more than one part of the brain.

This could be linked to the idea of the hyper-excitable brain, because the disinhibition could cause the brain to be more reactive to stimulation.

Furthermore, it could be the case that all of these theories are correct, and that synesthesia has more than one cause.

5) Brain-Imaging

Some neuroscientists have used brain-imaging technology, such as fMRI (Functional Magnetic Resonance Imaging) or PET (Positron Emitting Tomography) scanners to study the brains of synesthetes.

It is clear from these studies that a brain with synesthesia is substantially different from a brain without synesthesia. There is evidence that, for synesthetes who see colour when hearing words or sounds, certain parts of the visual cortex are more active than normal.

However, these technologies currently lack the level of detail that would prove or disprove the theories discussed above.

Chapter 4: Summary

- The brain has regions called 'cortices' which are dedicated to a certain function. For example, the visual cortex looks after sight.
- There are several theories about what causes synesthesia.
- Cross-Activation theory suggests that different cortices of the brain become connected together, producing blended senses.
- Some scientists argue that synesthetic brains are 'hyper excitable' and over-react to stimulus.
- Other scientists think that a process called 'inhibition' (which selects what feedback the brain consciously notices) is absent in synesthetes.
- It's possible that all of the above theories are true.
- Brain imaging shows that synesthetes' brains are different, but can't show enough detail to explain the causes of synesthesia.

Chapter 5) Have You Got Synesthesia?

In this chapter, we will look at how synesthesia is diagnosed: what the signs are, and who you should consult if you think you're affected by this condition.

1) The Symptoms of Synesthesia

On one hand, you might say that diagnosing synesthesia is simple: if you have one or more 'blended' senses, as described in Chapter 2, you could probably consider yourself a synesthete.

Many people self-diagnose in this way, because they don't feel the need to seek any treatment for the condition, and so don't need to bother with making an appointment with their doctor.

"I wouldn't even know where to go for a formal diagnosis! It was actually my partner who recognised it as synesthesia. I had never heard of it, yet anyone who is close to me is aware of my acute sense of smell. He had read about it a while back, and made the link to my description of how I experience smell." Melissa

However, medical professionals have to have more specific and exacting standards for making a diagnosis, especially for cases in which synesthesia is causing some level of suffering to the client, and will therefore require treatment.

It's worth noting first of all that, if a doctor thinks that a person might have synesthesia, they are unlikely to send them for an fMRI (Functional Magnetic Resonance Imaging) or PET (Positron Emitting Tomography) scan.

Although these brain imaging scans can usually detect unusual patterns in the brains of synesthetes, they are very expensive to conduct, and probably unnecessary. A person with synesthesia can usually tell their doctor enough information to get a good diagnosis, and there are also a range of tests that patients can complete themselves that make it clear not only whether they have synesthesia, but also what kind of synesthesia they have.

Try out our questionnaire below to see if you have synesthesia, and then read on to see what you should do about it.

"My synesthesia was identified when I was a child musician. It was how I communicated with music teachers and it actually helped me work through a kind of dyslexia, which also affected my ability to see symbols, like music notation, in the correct order. It took some time before it was 'realised' that I wasn't weird or stupid." Nicole

2) Questionnaire: Do you Have the Symptoms of Synesthesia?

1. Do you have unusual sensory experiences?
☐Yes
☐No

2. Can you choose whether or not you have your unusual sensory experiences?
☐Yes
☐No

3. Are your unusual sensory experiences the same every time you have them?
☐Yes
☐No

4. Are the unusual sensory experiences simple (e.g. basic colours, tastes or sounds instead of complex and detailed visions)?
☐Yes
☐No

5. Do one or more of your senses seem to be mixed with another sense?
☐Yes
☐No

6. Do your experiences leave a lasting impression?
☐Yes
☐No

7. Do you have an emotional response to your unusual sensory experiences?
☐Yes
☐No

If you answered yes to all of the questions, then you probably have synesthesia.

If you only answered yes to some of the questions, then it's not clear whether or not you have the condition. Take a look at the more detailed explanations below to get a better understanding of what we were looking for.

1. Do you have unusual sensory experiences?

The answer to this may well be, 'Of course I do! Otherwise I wouldn't be here in the first place!'

But the point is that, on a basic level, a synesthete must perceive at least one of their senses in a substantially different way to 'normal'.

2. Can you choose whether or not you have your unusual sensory experiences?

Synesthesia is an 'involuntary' experience – in other words, synesthetes have no control over whether or not they perceive the world in this way. So, if you can turn your experiences on and off, then you probably aren't a synesthete.

The important distinction here is that many people, particularly those working in the creative arts, can access a way of seeing the world that might be seen as synesthetic. They can imagine that sounds are colours, or that words have a taste. They can construct beautiful metaphors that blend several senses together (for example, 'the sea was sour today'). They may even be able to imagine these ideas to the extent that they can 'see' the colours that music creates or 'taste' the sourness of the sea.

However, unless those sensations arise without any effort or choosing, then that person is not a synesthete.

3. Are your unusual sensory experiences the same every time you have them?

Synesthesia is consistent – it is the same over and over again. This means that the same trigger always creates the same response. So, if you are a grapheme to colour synesthete, a certain letter might be yellow every time you see it; or Wednesday will always be red.

What's more, the colours won't switch; Wednesday won't sometimes be red and sometimes green. Neuroscientists have tested synesthetes over long periods of time, and they are certain that even very complex patterns of sensory blending stay exactly the same.

This criterion is designed to make the distinction between synesthesia, which is permanent, and more temporary conditions that may look similar at first glance. For example, drug use or a seizure could induce synesthesia-type symptoms.

Furthermore, in some cases people can 'train' themselves to have synesthesia-like symptoms (this may not be deliberate), and in these cases, the blended sensory perceptions tend not to have the complexity or consistency of neurological synesthesia – for example, they may report that 'c' is green in one test, and then that it is blue a year later.

4. Are the unusual sensory experiences simple?

This may sound like an odd question, but it's important to recognise the difference between synesthetic experiences and hallucinations.

In general, synesthetic experiences tend to be quite simple: for example, you are likely to hear one musical note or chord, or see a colour or pattern. If, instead, you heard a Welsh Male Voice Choir singing the Hallelujah Chorus, or saw a red dragon flying through the air, this would be unlikely to be a synesthetic experience.

The sensations experienced in synesthesia tend not to be complex because they are thought to come from very old parts of the brain in evolutionary terms. These brain areas fire off involuntarily when other senses are engaged, but they are not capable of high levels of detail or subtlety. Therefore, the experiences they produce will tend to be simple, although this doesn't mean to say that they aren't also intense and vivid. But they are often described as feeling 'natural' or 'elemental' by synesthetes.

If your experiences are more complex, this could be the result of a range of different conditions, or it could be the result of drug use. Unlike synesthesia, the presence of hallucinations can be a symptom of something serious, and so it's worth visiting your General Practitioner to discuss your experiences.

It is also worth doing this if you're not completely sure whether or not your unusual experiences are caused by synesthesia.

5. Have you considered the range of forms that synesthesia takes?

As we discussed in Chapter 2, synesthesia can take a wide range of forms. However, in popular understanding, synesthesia is often thought to just be seeing colours after input from other senses. This is because grapheme to colour synesthesia is by far the most common form of synesthesia, and so it tends to dominate the media coverage that the condition receives.

If you are having unusual sensory experiences, which entail 'feeling' or 'sensing' something that hasn't objectively happened, then you may have synesthesia, and it's worth taking a closer look at our list of the forms of synesthesia to see if there is anything you recognise.

Some types of synesthesia are easier to miss than others. For example, mirror touch synesthesia, in which someone gets a physical sensation from watching someone else touch something or – more often – get hurt, is not often recognised by people with the condition.

Similarly, forms of synesthesia that produce emotions are often tricky to recognise, and may be mistaken for other conditions such as depression. Like those that produce personification (projecting a character onto an object), people with the condition can assume that they have 'learned' to associate certain things with certain feelings.

However, if your perceptions fit the other criteria in this chapter, then you should consider whether this is synesthesia. Given that around 50 per cent of synesthetes have more than one type of synesthesia, the presence of other forms of the condition are a good sign, too.

6. Do your experiences leave a lasting impression?

Synesthesia tends to be highly memorable. When you think about it, it's unsurprising that it would stick in your mind!

Therefore, if you have an experience that feels like synesthesia, but you cannot remember ever having such an encounter before, it's unlikely that you have synesthesia, and could be experiencing something more temporary. On the contrary, people with neurological synesthesia (which results from the structure of the brain) will most likely be unable to remember a time when they did not experience the world in this way.

If your synesthesia-like experiences seem to have only appeared to emerge recently, it is once again a good idea to talk to your GP, because this can indicate a range of different problems, and it's sensible to get a check-up.

7. Do you have an emotional response to your unusual sensory experiences?

True synesthesia is 'laden with affect' as Cytowic put it when he outlined the features of synesthesia. This means that synesthetes have some sort of an emotional response to their experiences – they do not just feel neutrally about them and ignore them.

It's worth noting, though, that this does not necessarily mean a negative emotion. In fact, it's far more common for synesthetes to feel positive emotions, such as curiosity, wonder, joy, excitement and pleasure, when they have synesthetic experiences.

39

In fact, many synesthetes feel that their way of seeing the world is very special and enhances and sharpens their senses.

3) Visiting Your Doctor for Synesthesia

As I mentioned earlier, it's unlikely that your doctor will administer any physical tests for synesthesia. If you arrive in their office and list the symptoms of synesthesia, they may not even recognise them, because this may not be a condition that they are familiar with.

Even if you do come across a synesthesia-savvy doctor, the chances are that they will listen to your description of how you perceive the world, and simply say, 'Yes, that sounds like synesthesia to me,' and then politely show you out of their office.

This is because doctors are mainly only concerned with conditions that are causing suffering and discomfort, and, because synesthesia is generally harmless, if not a positive advantage to those who have it, your GP may not even enter it onto your medical records.

However, if you are experiencing synesthesia-like symptoms, especially if they seem to have started recently, or if you have read the list of diagnostic criteria in the last chapter and are not sure if they apply to your experiences, you should definitely visit your doctor. This is because some serious conditions – including epilepsy, brain tumours and schizophrenia – can have synesthesia-like symptoms, and so it's vital that you get a medical opinion to rule out any potential health problems.

The other reason that you should visit your doctor is if you think you have synesthesia, and it's causing you difficulties in everyday life. The majority of synesthetes don't experience any negative effects from the condition, but some do, and this can range from extreme aversions, negative emotions or feelings of disgust, which arise of synesthetic associations (such as certain words triggering an unbearable odour), or mirror touch synesthetes feeling high levels of discomfort from witnessing violent scenes on the television or in newspapers.

If this is the case, it's wise to ask your doctor for a referral to a neurologist, who is likely to have more expertise in your condition. However, as we will see in Chapter 7, treatment options are unfortunately limited and are in the early stages of development.

Some synesthetes report difficulties in communicating with their GPs about their synesthesia, either because the doctor doesn't know about the condition in the first place, and confuses it with mental illness, or because he or she doesn't understand the intensity with which synesthetes feel their blended senses, and so doesn't comprehend how serious problems arising from synesthesia can be.

If this is the case, here are some strategies that you could try:

Politely but firmly ask for a referral to a neurologist.
Asking directly in this way is often far more effective than waiting for the doctor to think of it.

Bring evidence.
Sometimes it pays to come prepared. If your doctor appears not to understand the condition, it may just be down to a simple gap in their knowledge. Do a little research on your particular form of synesthesia, and share your findings with your doctor. Keep it short and simple, and show them where they can get more information. Make sure that you emphasise that synesthesia is a condition that comes from the structure of the brain, rather than any emotional or learned behaviour.

Get a second opinion.
If your doctor is particularly unresponsive, don't be afraid to get a second opinion from another doctor- maybe even a third opinion if necessary. After all, this *is* a recognised condition, and any ignorance of that is their mistake.

Contact a synesthesia researcher.
An Internet search should help you to find a nearby university or hospital that is researching synesthesia. If you can find somewhere

where a researcher is interested in your particular form of synesthesia, so much the better. Most neuroscientists in the field will be happy to reply to a letter or email outlining your condition and asking for advice. You may like to ask them to recommend treatment routes or doctors who are sympathetic to your problems.

In fact, even if they are not experiencing any difficulties from their synesthesia, many synesthetes contact their most local research centre to volunteer for tests and trials. This can help them to gain more understanding of their condition, and to meet other people with similar experiences.

Of course, whether you choose to do this is entirely up to you!

4) Tests for Synesthesia

There is no one, standard test for synesthesia. This is because there are so many forms of synesthesia, and each of them have different sensory inputs and outputs. Some of these variations are so complex that it would be difficult to devise any one test.

As we already discussed, it is possible to use brain imaging such as fMRI or PET scans to diagnose synesthesia, but this is extremely expensive, and is rarely considered worth the expense or effort, as taking a case history is enough to diagnose most cases.

Where fMRI or PET scans are used, it tends to be for the purpose of research rather than diagnosis. For that reason, many synesthetes volunteer for medical research programmes, so that they can get access to scans of their own brain.

5) Questionnaires

Most researchers and doctors use a questionnaire to diagnose synesthesia, such as the one earlier in this chapter. Other such questionnaires can be found at:

http://www.sussex.ac.uk/synaesthesia/
(Sussex University)

or

http://brunel.ac.uk/~hsstnns/synaesthesia_RESEARCH.html
(Brunel University)

or

http://synesthete.org/pretest.php?action=register&remail=&semail
=&ch= (The Synesthesia Battery)

All of these questionnaires come from reputable universities and websites, and will be used to not only help you get a diagnosis, but will contribute to the body of knowledge on synesthesia. An Internet search will turn up a range of other questionnaires, too.

In the vast majority of cases, a simple questionnaire will give a medical professional all the evidence they need that a patient has synesthesia.

6) Online or Paper Tests

There are quite a few tests for synesthesia, and these tend to be used for research purposes rather than medical diagnosis.

However, they are useful when diagnosing children, or anyone who would struggle to answer the questions on a questionnaire. They also help to distinguish between people who have learned associations with certain stimuli (such as letters and numbers), and those who have synesthetic experiences due to the structure of their brain.

Unsurprisingly, there are as many tests for synesthesia as there are forms of the condition, and a synesthete will only 'pass' the tests designed specifically for their type of synesthesia.

A good test for the most common form of synesthesia, grapheme to colour synesthesia, is reproduced below.

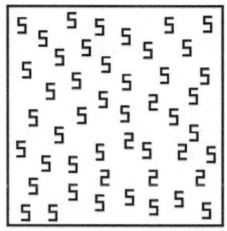

Source: http://youramazingbrain.org.uk

If you are not a synesthete, at first glance you will probably see many number fives arranged randomly. If you look closer, you may see that there are also some number twos, once again placed at random.

However, if you are a grapheme to colour synesthete, you will see an entirely different picture, because you will instantly recognise the twos and fives in different colours. Therefore, you will see a triangle of twos amongst a jumble of fives, somewhat like this:

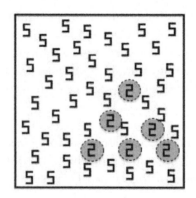

Even if you are not a synesthete, this test helps you to understand how someone with the condition will see the world completely differently, with no effort or thought needed.

Another interesting test covers a rare from of synesthesia- kinetics to sound. In this form, synesthetes will hear sounds when they see movement.

Take a look at the video here: http://youtu.be/o39TiACe4mw. If simply watching this makes you hear some kind of sound, whatever it is, you have this form of synesthesia. Don't forget that the sound has to emerge without any effort, and that it's likely to be a simple sound, such as a whirring or whooshing.

7) The Synesthesia Battery

One of the best and most comprehensive tests available is the Synesthesia Battery (Link shown above).

This is part of a research project by Dr David Eagleman, who is a neuroscientist and expert on synesthesia. People who already think or know they have synesthesia can log in online, and take the 'battery' (collection) of tests, that ascertain what kind of synesthesia they have and collect a greater depth of knowledge into the condition.

When you take the test, you have the choice to keep the results entirely to yourself, or to share your results with the research community so that they can gain a better understanding of synesthesia.

The aim of this project is to develop a series of 'standardised' tests for synesthesia, which means that all doctors and scientists across the world are using the same set of criteria to diagnose synesthesia. The test is available in nine languages.

If you would like to take part in the synesthesia battery, go to http://synesthete.org, where you will find a link to begin the battery of tests. If you are not sure whether or not you have synesthesia, take a short questionnaire on their homepage before you start.

Chapter 5 Summary: What Steps Should You Take?

If you think you have synesthesia, here's a decision tree to help you to decide what to do.

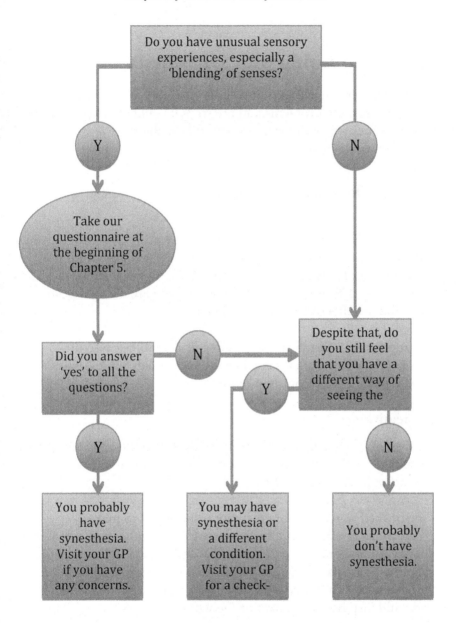

Chapter 6) Living with Synesthesia

In this chapter, we will look at what it's like to live with synesthesia – the benefits, the problems and the ways it could affect your career. The good news is that, for most synesthetes, the story is overwhelmingly positive.

1) The Benefits of Synesthesia

As we already know, synesthesia has an 'effect' on those who have it – it elicits an emotional response. For the vast majority of those with synesthesia, this is a positive one. They are fascinated and delighted by their way of seeing the world, and are often keen to share the benefits of having synesthesia.

It's impossible to list every single advantage here, because the experiences of synesthetes are so wide and varied, but let's take a look at the ten most common ones.

a. Creativity

As we will explore later in this chapter, synesthesia can be a huge advantage to those working in the creative arts, or simply those who use creativity to enhance their lives.

One of the foundations of creativity is the ability to make connections between different pieces of information, and to use that connection to generate something new and original. The brains of synesthetes are naturally wired to make these kinds of connections, and this means that they can think in ways that seem incredibly fresh and inspiring to the rest of the world.

Synesthetes excel in creating abstract or symbolic representations of real life. The paintings of Kandinsky, which we looked at in the introduction to this book, are a great example of this: he listened to music, and used his synesthetic experiences as a springboard to

48

create colourful, vibrant and original paintings. These, in turn, help non-synesthetes to imagine the world differently.

Another good example is the use of metaphors in writing. When writers make comparisons such as 'the sun was a juicy orange' or 'her voice sparkled,' they are using language in a synesthetic way, and yet creating images that non-synesthetes will immediately understand.

Music could be viewed as an abstract way of seeing the world, too. It often takes 'concrete' ideas, such as war or love, and uses those ideas to weave songs and symphonies that allow the audience to feel moods and emotions, without needing to use words.

Music is, in fact, a way that everyone can understand what it's like to have synesthesia. Most people will intuitively understand that minor chords 'feel' sad, and that major chords can, by contrast, 'feel' joyous or aggressive. Similarly, most people will find that certain instruments have a haunting or melancholy tone (this is often true for wind instruments), and that others are naturally more boisterous (brass instruments, for example). This gives us a glimpse into the world of the synesthete: two unconnected things become connected, and our understanding is natural and instant.

"As a singer I'd say it's an asset, as it's an added facet of the way I interpret and perform music. I think if I woke one day and didn't hear colours, I'd be a bit sad. Likewise, if I sang some Wagner and didn't see the colour wash, I'd probably miss it." Nicole

Synesthetes working in the creative arts often make use of their intuitive understanding, creating work that helps non-synesthetes to make fresh connections, too.

b. Memory

Synesthesia is strongly associated with enhanced memory skills. In fact, some synesthetes are capable of performing extraordinary feats of memory.

Daniel Tammet, for example, has been recorded reciting all the digits of the mathematical constant pi from memory, up to over 22,000 decimal places! For those of us who can only recall 3.14, that's extraordinarily impressive.

If we dig a little deeper into this phenomena, we can identify two ways in which synesthesia may help memory. First of all, the experiences of synesthesia make everyday things more memorable. Daniel Tammet is a good example of this: for him, every number up to 10,000 has its own colour and texture, as well as a physical sensation attached to it. Therefore, when he tries to remember a long number, he is naturally using the kind of technique that experts recommend for enhancing memory. A number 23 is much more memorable if it is green and fuzzy.

Neuroscientists also think that the enhanced memory of synesthetes may be connected to the fact that the gene for synesthesia sits on the same area of the same chromosome as autism. This could mean that synesthetes are able to store memories in the same way as autistic savants, another group renowned for impressive memory skills.

c. Sensitivity

The senses of synesthetes are not just blended – they may also be heightened.

Some studies have suggested that synesthetes show increased sensitivity in the senses linked to their condition. For example, those people who see colours as a result of synesthesia tend to be able to better understand subtle differences between colours. Similarly, people with mirror touch synesthesia seem to have a more fine tuned sense of touch.

These levels of sensitivity can be hugely useful in the jobs that synesthetes do; for example, a massage therapist may benefit from the skills that come with mirror touch synesthesia.

d. Mathematical abilities

Certain types of synesthesia seem to lead to enhanced mathematical abilities.

This may, in part, be linked to the ability to memorise numbers, due to numbers being associated with texture, pattern, taste or colour. Put quite simply, for synesthetes with these kinds of synesthesia, numbers may simply be more unique and memorable.

However, another form of synesthesia called 'spatial sequence synesthesia' is also linked to enhanced mathematical abilities. In this form, synesthetes see sequences and numbers at fixed points in space. For example, the numbers one to ten may form a line projecting outwards, or a spiral.

This means that these individuals have an entirely different relationship with equations to the rest of the world: they can see them arrayed before their eyes, and it's easier for them to see interconnections between different parts of the equation.

The enhanced memory skills mentioned in the last point may also contribute to a better understanding of mathematics.

e. Empathy

Mirror touch synesthesia can be seen as an extreme form of empathy. People with this condition feel sensations that they see other people receiving: so they may see somebody cut their finger and experience some form of sensation themselves. This could be anything from a vague tingle to a feeling of pain identical to the person who has actually sustained the injury.

For some synesthetes, therefore, it is possible to feel high levels of empathy for other people and animals. These synesthetes don't have to use their imagination to put themselves in someone else's shoes; they are in their shoes.

This can be hugely beneficial in everyday relationships, such as friendships and parenting, and for professional roles such as counselling or even sales.

f. Attention

Synesthetes tend to be unable to ignore their condition; in fact, they are quite likely to find it fascinating. When a synesthetic experience happens, the synesthete's attention is drawn very strongly to it – some people describe this as 'zooming in.'

So, for example, if you have grapheme colour synesthesia, and associate letters with colours, you may find that you focus very strongly on any written materials, which can lead to you remembering it better afterwards, or simply being able to analyse it in more detail.

This means synesthesia can be a huge advantage to people who need to understand their work in a great deal of detail, for example- accountants or editors.

g. Planning

Some synesthetes can visualise units of time as having a specific location in space. So, for example, the months of the year may form an oval. One synesthete told me:

"I visualise time in decades of different colours and in a helical construction." Sheila

This ability to actually 'see' time can be enormously helpful in planning, because synesthetes can get a better mental picture of how a project will pan out across months and years.

This can make this form of synesthesia hugely beneficial to project managers or wedding planners.

h. 3-D thinking

Richard Cytowic, in his first list of the features of synesthesia, thought that all synesthetes were 'localizers,' meaning that they saw their synesthetic experiences projected out into the real world, rather than in their heads (he called this 'spatially extended').

Later neuroscientists found that this wasn't true of all synesthetes, but for some it can be a highly useful trait. This kind of '3-D thinking' can be hugely useful for architects and engineers, who otherwise have to rely on making models and complex diagrams to get a full picture of their planned projects.

This kind of ability may also help physicists and mathematicians when they're solving problems related to mechanics.

i. All Senses Enhanced

Some research suggests that synesthetes don't only benefit from extra abilities in the senses affected by their synesthesia, but that all their senses are enhanced to some extent, and that they can more easily make connections between their senses.

This may mean that synesthetes are 'super-sensers' who are particularly adept at observing and analyzing the outside world. It is thought that this trait has survived in the human population because the genes would have been beneficial for man throughout time. For example, synesthetes would have made excellent hunters because all their senses are so finely tuned.

j. Fascination

One of the greatest gifts of synesthesia is the fascination it gives to those who have it. This can be an enormous pleasure, drawing synesthetes into the present moment when their experiences occur.

Some synesthetes say that they feel especially calm when they are having synesthetic experiences. Others simply feel that they have an amusing extra skill.

Whatever the level of interest, it seems clear that synesthesia can be a source of pride and entertainment for those who have it.

2) Problems Associated with Synesthesia

Synesthesia is not generally considered to be a 'disease' in the way that many other genetically-inherited neurological conditions are. Compared to its genetic cousins, epilepsy and autism, its effects are mostly mild, if not positively beneficial.

However, the experience of synesthesia isn't without complications, which range from minor irritations with the experiences that synesthesia brings, to difficulties and disadvantages that make everyday life difficult. A minority of synesthetes will even seek treatment for the condition.

For these people, the assumption that synesthesia is always an advantage can be extremely frustrating, and so it's important to point out that synesthetes need treating with sensitivity. They are often bombarded with curious questions when people find out that they have the condition, and although many are delighted to talk about their synesthesia, some will be less enamoured with their experiences.

One group who can find synesthesia particularly difficult is young people, particularly teenagers. At an age when it's common to become self-conscious about being different, synesthesia can be highly embarrassing and awkward, with young people feeling that they get 'caught out' by letting on that they see the world in this special way.

In addition, the process of coming to realise that your synesthetic experiences are unusual can, in itself, be an unsettling time for children, who may have anxieties that they have a 'disability' or that they are 'weird'. Without support, some children will misunderstand their synesthetic experiences, and attribute them to the wrong causes, for example supernatural forces.

Therefore, if you have a child with synesthesia, it's important to encourage them to talk about their experiences, and to provide them with accurate information. It can be worth talking to their school to ensure that there is a full understanding of the situation, and to put strategies into place that deal with any specific difficulties that your child might have.

Children aside, synesthetes report a range of problems and issues that can arise from their condition. Here are the most common:

a. Bias

Many forms of synesthesia create sensations that are enjoyable or unpleasant for the synesthete. For example, if hearing sounds leads you to taste distinct flavours, it's possible that some of these flavours will be either delicious or disgusting. Similarly, people whose synesthesia leads to personification (sensing a character from an object) can take strong likes or dislikes to objects because of their projected personality.

The effect of this can be very difficult to handle. This is because the synesthete may experience a 'bad' taste in response to an everyday sound, or one that is perfectly pleasant. Or, they may take an intense dislike to a certain letter or number, because their personification creates a nasty character.

This can mean that synesthetes find it very difficult to assess and judge things objectively. A passage of music that is crucial for an examination at school, for example, may be so imbued with positive or negative flavours that the synesthete cannot write an unbiased essay on the subject. Or a person could find it difficult to pay their bills because of an aversion to a certain number, which comes from its 'personality' being unpleasant in some way.

Therefore, synesthetes often find that the biases that emerge from their condition can have a negative impact on everyday life.

b. Overload

Imagine how this feels: you walk down the street to pick up a few groceries. Every shop sign and poster glows in multiple colours. The voices of people drift by, each of them making you taste a different flavour. The colourful window displays trigger a range of noises to sound in your ears.

This is how a very simple shopping trip can feel to synesthetes, particularly those with multiple types of synesthesia. Many complain of encountering 'sensory overload' at least sometimes, and for some synesthetes, this overwhelming barrage of sensations is an everyday occurrence, making even the most ordinary activity feel totally exhausting and putting them on edge.

And, of course, it's impossible to 'switch off' synesthesia. It's constant and inescapable. What's more, most of the ways that non-synesthetes relax offer no escape to some synesthetes – for example, watching television or listening to music can create a cacophony of extra experiences that make it very hard to rest.

c. Spatial awareness

There are two common spatial problems that seem to occur in a large number of synesthetes:

Left-right confusion, which means that some synesthetes find it almost impossible to associate the words 'left' and 'right' with those physical directions. This can make driving tests very difficult, as well as being given a whole range of basic directions for finding things.

Poor sense of direction. This does not affect all synesthetes, but many find it difficult to navigate when driving or walking, and can easily get lost in unfamiliar environments.

These spatial difficulties appear to be linked to the genetic basis of synesthesia. It's likely that both left-right confusion and a poor sense of direction is found in the same area of the brain as synesthesia, and so gets bundled into the condition.

d. Mathematical abilities

We already discussed how synesthesia can enhance the mathematical abilities of those with the condition. It is unfortunately also true that, for many synesthetes, mathematics is unusually difficult.

Once again, this can be due to the synesthete becoming overwhelmed by the information they receive from a simple sum; after all, numbers contain extra experiences and information for many synesthetes. It can also be due to bias and aversions created by synesthetic perceptions, making people feel more drawn to some numbers than others.

But one researcher, M. J. Dixon, showed that synesthetes need to be able to do maths in a synesthetic manner. They found that a synesthete who associates numbers with colours will do better if the solution to an equation is colour-coded to match the person's synesthetic expectations. If, however, the colours clash (and think how colourful many textbooks are these days), they were less likely to get the correct answer.

Therefore, synesthetes may be at a disadvantage in mathematics because textbooks are not designed with their needs in mind.

e. Uncertainty

Synesthetic experiences feel so natural that it can be difficult to tell the difference between synesthesia and real life. One synesthete that I interviewed, who experiences sounds as odours, explained that:

"Sometimes I get a whiff of something bad, and I'm not sure whether it's something I should investigate or whether it's just a sound I'm hearing." Joanne

As this example shows, the world can be a confusing place for some synesthetes. Some can become anxious because they are concerned that they will not be able to tell the difference between the real and the imaginary. This could lead to potential embarrassment, but it could also be dangerous, if, for example a synesthete fails to realise that a burning smell is a real fire.

f. Over-sensitivity

Yet another flip-side of the benefits of synesthesia: those enhanced senses can actually be over-sensitive.

For synesthetes, it can be hard to switch off or ignore the senses, because they are so well-attuned. Therefore, the smell of food, which is pleasant for most people, can be cloying to a highly sensitive nose. Music can be too loud at a low volume; or the slightest flaw in pitch or harmony can rattle the nerves. Bright colours can tip over from being cheerful into being an assault on the eyes.

"I'm often saying: can you smell that? And no one around me can smell anything. It means that certain smells I find intolerable and make me feel nauseous. I experience it more vividly than other people.
Sometimes it works to the contrary where some smells have a similar pattern so I find them hard to distinguish and some vivid smells difficult to name! I'm always stumped with jasmine, which is arguably one of the most recognisable smells. It is beautiful, yet to me I don't connect the smell to the plant." Joanne

It's also common for synesthetes to choose very neutral colours in their home and for their clothes, as they are trying to create environments that are as un-stimulating as possible, in an attempt to gain some sanctuary from the outside world.

The over-sensitivity can also take place in emotional matters, where synesthetes can find themselves too conscious of other people's feelings and attitudes, leaving them feeling overwhelmed by their empathy.

g. Visual obstruction

Some forms of synesthesia generate visions of colour, text or pattern which appear to float before the eyes, or which hang around people and objects as 'auras'.

This means that some synesthetes complain that their vision is actually obscured at times, and that it is unpredictable when this will happen.

For highly sensitive synesthetes, this can make driving or operating machinery dangerous. Some say that the visions intensify with more intense stimuli – so, for example, hearing a fire alarm will set of very dense visualisations, whereas normal levels of noise, such as the television or washing machine, will only produce lighter, more manageable visions.

For some synesthetes, this problem is so severe that they are unable to drive at all, or carry out many jobs, because of the risks to their safety. This is rare, but there is a much larger group of synesthetes for whom visual disturbance is a constant, nagging nuisance over which they have no control.

h. Mirror touch

As we already know, mirror touch synesthesia means that you can 'feel' physical sensations that are happening to other people – your brain is literally 'mirroring' the experiences. This tends to be more acute for unpleasant sights, so violence, pain or illness will trigger the synesthetic effects for most mirror touch synesthetes.

"When I watch something violent in a film or on TV, I feel everything. It doesn't hurt, but I get a sort of dull tingle in the part of my body that I saw get hurt. I can't help myself; I have to wince and put my hand on it. It feels really uncomfortable. The worst for me is vomiting. If I see someone being sick, I'm sick too. I just can't help it." Chris

This is rarely a pleasant experience. Even those with mild forms of the condition can feel constantly physically invaded by what they see. If they observe people kissing or hugging, it can be pleasant although a little annoying at times. But watching television or opening the newspaper can be a minefield, fraught with the risk of seeing something that will become mapped out of their own body.

For those synesthetes with more severe responses, mirror touch synesthesia can be agony. In these very rare cases, a synesthete will feel actual pain when they witness someone else's pain, and this can be extremely intense.

People with this form of synesthesia can feel very isolated, as they have to carefully avoid many forms of media, and so lack the same cultural references as the people around them.

3) Synesthesia and Creativity

Synesthesia and the creative arts are so intertwined that they merit a whole chapter. Although not all synesthetes would identify themselves as being creative, many do, and their unique perceptive abilities mean that they have a great deal to offer in terms of original thought and fresh ways of seeing.

Here, we will look in more detail about three key ways in which synesthesia has contributed to the creative arts: music, literature and visual art.

Synesthesia and Music

Synesthesia and music often go hand-in-hand. For synesthetes, hearing music can trigger a wide variety of senses, including colour, pattern, taste and smell. This means that some synesthetes have a depth of experience when they listen to music that far transcends anything that non-synesthetes can imagine.

Popular music abounds with synesthetic references, especially to colour. The blues is a phrase we're so familiar with that it's easy to miss how synesthetic it is to describe a mood using a colour.

One famous contemporary musician with synesthesia is the rock artist John Mayer. Mayer sees music as colour, and has written about how he relates to his hero, Jimi Hendrix, who also reported synesthesia-like experiences.

Hendrix is on record as claiming that he didn't play notes, but colours. However, he never spoke about synesthesia per se, and may

60

not even have been aware that the condition existed. He was also an enthusiastic user of LSD, and so it's not entirely clear whether he was a genuine synesthete, or whether he had simply experienced temporary synesthesia-like effects from his drug use.

Many other pop and rock musicians have (or seem to have) synesthesia, including Billy Joel, Stevie Wonder, Tori Amos and Mary J Blige. Analysis of historical texts and diaries by historians and neuroscientists has suggested that many classical composers also showed synesthesia symptoms.

Franz Liszt, for example, famously asked an orchestra to play, 'a little bluer, please! This tone type requires it!'

Nikolai Rimsky-Korsakov documented his synesthesia in great detail. He associated each musical pitch with a different colour, so that E was sapphire blue, G was brownish gold and A was rosy. He also experimented with projecting colours onto a screen behind the orchestra during a few of his concerts, so that the audience could see what he saw when they heard his music. However, this was largely ignored by the assembled people.

Perhaps the most famous composer of all, Ludvig van Beethoven, is thought to have had synesthesia. He is known to have described certain keys as colours – for example, D minor was orange and B minor was black.

Therefore, it seems that synesthesia has influenced some of the most important people in the history of music. However, it is also a source of great curiosity to non-synesthetes, who have often referred to synesthesia when making music. Lady Gaga has talked about synesthesia in one of her most famous songs, and a simple Internet search reveals a fascination with synesthesia amongst the musical community.

You can even download a programme called 'Synesthesia Piano' that allows you to learn piano using ideas based on synesthesia. The learner is encouraged to associate certain notes with colours. And perhaps the most famous electronic drum-pad is called the Synesthesia Mandala Drum.

It's clear that synesthesia is something that musicians want to be associated with, even if they do not have it themselves.

Synesthesia and Art

We have already discussed Wassily Kandinsky's synesthesia – he is perhaps the most famous artist to have the condition because his paintings are such pure expressions of shape and colour. Kandinsky was also fascinated by the condition himself, and related it to his spiritual beliefs in theosophy, thinking that the most pure expressions of synesthesia would take him to a higher plane of existence.

David Hockney is perhaps the most famous living artist with synesthesia, and his approach is a great deal more down-to-earth! He sees colours when he hears music, and has used this to inform the numerous stage sets that he has designed over his career. However, he claims that he does not let his synesthesia influence his paintings.

It is also thought that Vincent van Gogh was a synesthete, although this is unconfirmed. In one of his letters to Theo van Gogh in 1881, he appears to describe a form of synesthesia opposite to David Hockney's: he hears the work of different artists as sound.

Just as musicians have sought to have synesthesia-like experiences even if they don't have the condition themselves, many visual artists are fascinated by the visual effects of synesthesia.

For example, a Danish designer called Jeppe Carlsen has created a video game called Synesthesia, which aims to reproduce the experience of being a synesthete though many colourful screens.

Synesthesia in Poetry and Prose

It's unsurprising that many writers have also been synesthetes.

Vladimir Nabokov, for example, wrote extensively about his experiences as a synesthete in his autobiography, Speak Memory. He called his synesthesia 'coloured hearing' but on closer inspection it appears to be more akin to phoneme to colour synesthesia, as it focuses on the sounds that make up words. This is suggested by the fact that Nabokov's synesthesia appeared to distinguish between the same letters in different languages.

However, he also seems to get a sensation of texture from his synesthetic associations, as you can see from this fascinating passage:

"The long a of the English alphabet...has more of the tint of weathered wood, but a French a evokes polished ebony. This black group also includes hard g (vulcanised rubber) and r (a sooty rag being ripped). Oatmeal n, noodle-limp l, and the ivory-backed hand mirror of o take care of the whites...Passing on to the blue group there is steely x, thundercloud z, and huckleberry k." Vladimir Nabokov

Nabokov appeared to have inherited his synesthesia from his mother, and he passed it onto his son.

Other famous authors with synesthesia include Joanne Harris, Orhan Pamuk and Julie Myerson.

Many poems contain synesthesia-like images, to the extent that synesthesia is a standard term in poetry criticism. The technique of using one sense to describe another is very appealing to poets, who use it to inject vividness and interest into their work. A famous example is Keats' phrase, 'sunburnt mirth' in Ode to a Nightingale, but the use of synesthesia has become increasingly popular with contemporary poets.

In recent years, the interest of the creative world in synesthesia has led to a number of novels featuring characters with the condition. For example, Clare Morrall's 'Astonishing Splashes of Colour' is an in-depth portrayal of the life of an eccentric synesthete, and Dean Koontz's 'Intensity' deals with similar themes.

Chapter 6 Summary

- There are many benefits to synesthesia, and many consider it to be a gift.
- However, for a minority of synesthetes, synesthesia will make everyday life challenging.
- It's important to recognise that everyone's experience of synesthesia is different, and to be sensitive when speaking to people about their condition.
- Synesthesia has informed many of the creative arts, including music, visual art and writing.

Chapter 7) Treatment Options for
Synesthesia

The vast majority of synesthetes will never want to treat their synesthesia, either because it's a wholly positive experience, or because it's only a minor irritation. However, some synesthetes will need to seek treatment because their condition is having a negative effect on their life.

We outline the options.

1) Problems with Treating Synesthesia

For those synesthetes searching for a treatment for synesthesia, the experience can be very disheartening.

There are very few treatments for synesthesia at all, and this is partly because scientists still do not fully understand the condition, and partly because there is so little demand for a treatment or cure.

There are also a huge body of synesthetes and neuroscientists who strongly feel that synesthesia should not be treated, because it is a gift and a wonderful way of seeing the world. These people argue that their condition should be nurtured and understood, and that no synesthete should try to change or get rid of their synesthesia at all.

This offers little help to the minority of synesthetes for whom the condition causes suffering, though. It's important to acknowledge that some synesthetes simply do not feel that their experiences are a blessing. And, equally, we should never seek to suggest that we should treat synesthesia just because it is 'different'. Synesthesia should only be treated in patients who feel that they need treatment: it's a personal choice, rather than a blanket strategy.

For people who are having minor difficulties with their synesthesia, or who have only just learned that they have it and are unsure what that means, the first port of call may be talking to other synesthetes. There are many chat-boards and support groups for synesthetes online, or alternatively, the resources section at the back of this book contains information on national associations for synesthetes.

Talking about your synesthesia with other people can help to relieve anxiety and to share experiences with other people who will understand exactly what you mean. The online communities are generally very friendly and helpful, and are happy to answer questions or offer suggestions, tips or advice for managing the more difficult aspects of being a synesthete.

What follows is a brief summary of treatment options- should you still feel that you need extra help; it should be emphasised, however, that there is little medical evidence that anything works particularly well, and so any treatment you undertake should be in consultation with your doctor.

You will most likely need to try out a few solutions and decide what seems to work for you personally.

Medication

There are no drug therapies available for synesthesia.

Occasionally, doctors have prescribed anti-depressants or anti-anxiety medication, but this is generally to treat the patient's reaction to their synesthesia, rather than the synesthesia itself. Similarly, sleeping tablets are sometimes offered.

With any of these drugs, it's not desirable to be using them in the long-term, and so it's wise to consider other strategies, such as talking therapies, to compliment any medication.

Talking Therapies

Synesthesia is not a mental illness, and cannot be cured by treating it as such.

However, spending time with a counsellor or psychotherapist can help synesthetes to find strategies to manage their condition, and to come to terms with any negative feelings they have around it.

Some synesthetes would even benefit from occupational therapy or coaching, which would support them to develop ways of working around their condition, so that the negative effects of their synesthesia feel more manageable. This may involve anything from changing their environment to choosing work that draws on the positive aspects of synesthesia.

Hypnosis

Hypnotherapy is the process of putting people into a very relaxed state so that they are receptive to suggestions. There is often a prejudice against using hypnotherapy, because most people have seen stage hypnotists humiliating people for entertainment, or think that it is a 'quack' therapy. However, hypnotherapy has been scientifically proven to be safe and effective for a variety of problems.

Some people also fear losing control when under hypnosis. In actual fact (and unlike the people you see being hypnotised on television), being under hypnosis is more like being in a very light sleep than being completely unconscious. You will most likely remember what happened during your session, and will feel as though you have the choice to finish the session at any time.

Neuroscientists report some success with using hypnosis to alleviate any problems caused by synesthesia. It is thought that hypnosis can help to remove negative associations, and to gain a better understanding of exactly how the senses are blended.

It's vital to choose a hypnotherapist who fully understands synesthesia, and who also understands the nature of the work that can be done. Be extremely wary of any hypnotherapist who claims that they can 'cure' synesthesia, or who doesn't understand the neurological basis of the condition.

Remember: it's perfectly reasonable to ask questions, and any therapist who is angry or uncomfortable with this probably isn't the right person for you.

Alternative Approaches

It's important to note that there's no scientific evidence that supports the use of any alternative therapy for the treatment of synesthesia.

Yet, many synesthetes use alternative remedies, such as acupuncture, reiki and reflexology to alleviate the negative symptoms of synesthesia. There is certainly no harm in doing this, and it may work for you. Choose a therapy that you're drawn to, and speak to the therapist about your aims for the treatment.

In some alternative communities, the symptoms of synesthesia are seen as sings of spiritual awareness. It's occasionally explained as seeing chakras or auras, of being the beginning of a shamanic experience, for example. If these beliefs fit with your own, then it can be a wonderful way of acknowledging and honouring your unique way of seeing the world.

Beware, though, of any spiritual or religious belief that claims that your synesthesia is a sign of possession or other evil. This most likely comes from ignorance of what causes synesthesia, and you should not be made to feel as though your condition is a character flaw.

Equally, if you are not comfortable with undertaking therapies that are not part of mainstream science, then feel free to avoid them.

2) Future Treatments – Gene Therapy

There is currently no cure for synesthesia.

Research into gene therapy is ongoing for a range of conditions, and it is possible that, in the future, it will be possible to 'switch off' the gene for synesthesia. However, it is likely that this will emerge from research into treating the conditions that share a chromosome with synesthesia – epilepsy and autism. This means that gene therapy for synesthesia will probably be low on the list of priorities.

What does this mean in practice? Well, gene therapies use drugs or biological agents (such as viruses) to replace unwanted genes with preferred ones. If a gene therapy were developed for synesthesia, it would possibly have to be given to parents trying to conceive, so that their future children would not have synesthesia.

It is unlikely that gene therapy would have much effect on adults who already have synesthesia. This is because the genes have already done their work in determining how the brain develops, and replacing the genes as an adult is unlikely to change this. However, it may give hope to families who have a history of severe forms of synesthesia.

This treatment is controversial, though. Some object on religious or ethical grounds, arguing that doctors should not 'play god' with the genetic makeup of people, and that gene therapies seek to erase disability and difference from our society, not appreciating the huge benefits that this diversity brings.

Others argue that gene therapies would only be used to prevent suffering, and that it is no different to using drugs to treat other conditions.

A further problem for those seeking to treat synesthesia with gene therapies is that, although it is passed on from parent to child, it is not always the same form of synesthesia that appears. So, for example, a parent with grapheme to colour synesthesia may have a child with colour to music synesthesia.

What's more, everyone experiences and interprets their synesthesia differently. This means that a parent who feels overwhelmed by multiple forms of synesthesia may have a child who adores being a synesthete. Therefore, parents could potentially employ gene therapy to get rid of a beneficial and pleasant condition.

Finally, over-use of gene therapy could mean that synesthesia disappears from the population, which would be a huge loss.

Any discussion of this is purely theoretical at the moment, though. When gene therapies do emerge, each individual will have to judge what they want to do based on their own needs and experiences.

Chapter 7 Summary

- There is no cure for synesthesia.
- Treatment options are limited, and you may need to try out a few approaches before you get the result you want.
- Hypnotherapy is generally seen by neuroscientists as the most useful treatment.
- There may be gene therapies in the future.
- Many synesthetes would object to the very idea of a treatment or cure.
- If your symptoms are causing suffering, you should make up your own mind as to what therapies to pursue.

Chapter 8) Resources

In this section, you will find a list of resources to help you to learn more about synesthesia, and to meet others who have the same experiences as you. This includes websites, books and membership associations, as well as a selection of materials that feature synesthesia in the creative arts.

1) Groups and Associations

UK Synesthesia Association

http://www.uksynaesthesia.com
Provides information and support for synesthetes, including a newsletter and conferences. Aims to connect synesthetes with the academic community.

American Synesthesia Association

http://www.synesthesia.info
Offers information to synesthetes and scientists, and raises money to support research into synesthesia.

The Canadian Synesthesia Association

http://synesthesiacanada.com
Aims to raise awareness of synesthesia as a condition, and lobbies for further recognition and research. Works to create a community of synesthetes in Canada.

Synesthesia Meetup Groups

http://synesthesia.meetup.com
A site for people who want to meet others who share their experiences.

Synesthesia Facebook Group

https://www.facebook.com/pages/Synesthesia
This is a space where synesthetes share experiences and ideas. It also seems to be a portal through which researchers contact synesthetes for research.

2) Information Websites

Mixed Signals

http://www.mixsig.net
A good source of information on synesthesia, including a chat-board and events calendar for synesthetes.

DaySyn

http://www.daysyn.com
This is compiled by Sean Day, the president of the American Synesthesia Association, and gathers together resources on synesthesia, including some great videos. It includes the best available list on the frequency of various forms of synesthesia, which is updated regularly.

Synesthesia Down Under

http://synesthesia.com.au
This Australian site provides a forum, links to researchers and other information.

Synesthesia for Kids

http://faculty.washington.edu/chudler/syne.html
This is an information page aimed at introducing young people to synesthesia. However, some of the writing is quite sophisticated, so it's probably best for older kids.

The Synesthetic Experience

http://web.mit.edu/synesthesia/www/synesthesia.html
This is a page that gathers together resources on synesthesia, with useful first-hand accounts and films for teachers.

3) Tests for Synesthesia

The Synesthesia Battery

http://www.synesthete.org
This is the most comprehensive test, and is set to become the standard diagnostic for synesthesia. It assumes that you already have synesthesia, and seeks to assess what form you have, using both visual tests and questionnaires.

Synesthesia Test

http://www.synesthesiatest.org
A short online questionnaire that will help to determine whether you're a synesthete.

Sussex University

http://www.sussex.ac.uk/synaesthesia/
A questionnaire developed by Sussex University.

Brunel University

http://brunel.ac.uk/~hsstnns/synaesthesia_RESEARCH.html
A questionnaire developed by Brunel University.

4) Books on Synesthesia

Neuroscience:

The following are studies of the condition. They may be quite academic in tone, but they are also fascinating accounts of the neuroscience and experiences of synesthesia.

Wednesday is Indigo Blue by Richard Cytowic and David Eagleman (2011, MIT Press)

The Man Who Tasted Shapes by Richard Cytowic (2003, MIT Press)

Synesthesia: A Union of the Senses by Richard Cytowic (1989, Springer)

The Frog Who Croaked Blue: Synesthesia and the Mixing of the Senses by Jamie Ward (2008, Routledge)

The Tell-Tale Brain: Unlocking the Mystery of Human Nature by V S Ramachandran (2012, Windmill)

Incognito: The Secret Lives of the Brain by David Eagleman (2012, Canongate)

The Oxford Handbook of Synesthesia by Julia Simner and Edward M Hubbard (2013, Oxford University Press)

I Is An Other by James Geary (2012, Harper Perennial)

Memoir:

These books are written by synesthetes, recounting their experiences.

Born on a Blue Day by Daniel Tammet (2007, Hodder Paperbacks)

The Shaking Woman or a History of My Nerves by Siri Hustvedt (2011, Sceptre)

The Alphabet in Colour by Vladimir Nabokov and Jean Holabird

Eccentricity by Anie Knipping (Amazon Media)

Blue Cats and Chartreuse Kittens by Patricia Lynne Duffy (2002, Owl Books)

Novels Featuring Synesthetes:

A Mango-Shaped Space by Wendy Maas (2005, Little Brown)

Astonishing Splashes of Colour by Clare Morrall (2013, Sceptre)

The Particular Sadness of Lemon Cake by Aimee Bender (2011, Windmill)

Intensity by Dean Koontz (1996, Headline

Index

CPSIA information can be obtained
at www.ICGtesting.com
Printed in the USA
BVOW06s1915030817

491076BV00017B/137/P